Cancer: A Story of Death and Survival

Cancer: A Story of Death and Survival

By: Guy Rausch

Table of Contents

<u>Forward</u>

This is a story about cancer, what it is, the treatments for it and who it effects. I also shared with you how cancer has affected me personally. I shared how cancer whittle my dad down to nothing before taking his life but it spared my son's life.

<u>Dedication</u>

I want to dedicate this book to God first and foremost and to all the organizations and people out there that helped us through these hard times.

Chapter One

Cancer is a very, very nasty disease. It so extremely hard to see a love one is diagnosed with it. There is nothing you can do but watch them whittle down to practically nothing. The only thing you can honestly do is pray to God that he will work through the doctor to cure our love one.

As I am writing this book I started to wonder just how many types of cancer are there. I decided get on the internet and do a search. I went to my google search bar and typed in how many types of cancer are there. When the results came up I scrolled down the list and I came across this statement, *"Cancer is not just one disease but many diseases. There are more than 100 different types of cancer. Most cancers are named for the organ or type of cell in which they start - for example, cancer that begins in the colon is called colon cancer; cancer that begins in melanocytes of the skin is called melanoma (Mar. 7, 2014)."*

After reading this statement I thought to myself that is a lot. That got me to thinking just how many people die from cancer each year. So, once again I did a search in my google search engine and typed in how many people die each year from cancer. The results popped up and I started looking at the results when I came across this statement, *"Currently, 7.6 million people die from cancer worldwide every year (Feb. 4, 2013)."*

I read this statement and my mouth dropped open and I thought to myself that is an extremely lot of people that die from cancer each year. I knew it was going to be a lot but honestly I did think for the life of me that it would be that much. WOW!!! I truly thought that my eyes were playing tricks on me. I cannot get over the fact that **7.6 million people worldwide die each year from cancer!!!** Did you see what I just what I typed take a moment and look at it again. I cannot wrap my brain around those numbers.

According to a website I found which is sponsored by the American Cancer Society has to say about how cancer works. *"The body is made up of trillions of normal healthy cells. Cancer starts when something causes changes in a normal cell. This cancer cell then grows out of control and makes more cancer cells. Each type of cancer affects the body in different ways. If cancer is not treated, it can spread and affect the rest of your body*

Now you know why I made the statement that cancer is a very, very nasty disease. I am highly surprised that a cure hasn't been developed yet. There are a lot of organizations out there that are collecting money to help find a cure. There are some wonderful organizations like the American Cancer Society; Cops Fighting Cancer; Children's Cancer Research Fund; American Childhood Cancer Foundation; Stand Up To Cancer; Network For Good; Alex's Lemonade Stand Foundation and the list goes on and on.

These organizations raise hundreds of millions of dollars that they use to help cancer patients and fund research for a cure for cancer. That is a whole lot of money and it seems like it is taking forever for any of these organizations to find a cure.

It is heartwarming to know that some many people donated to these cancer organizations to the point that they are able to raise that kind of money. That is truly amazing that the amount of money that is being raised to find a cure for cancer. I hope with these organizations raising this kind of money that a cure will be found very soon.

Chapter Two

There are several treatments for cancer depending on the type. How far along it is? After researching it and this is what I found out. *"Surgery, chemotherapy and radiation are the most common types of cancer treatment. Surgery is often the first treatment option if the tumor can be taken out of the body. Sometimes only part of the tumor can be removed. Radiation, chemotherapy, or both might be used to shrink the tumor before or after surgery (Feb. 27, 2015)."*

Surgery is where they take the patient into the operating room open them up and go in and cut all the cancer out of their body. With this treatment they can only hope that they are able to get it all and mostly all the time the doctor says they got it all but that doesn't mean that the cancer won't come back.

Then there is chemotherapy. *"Chemotherapy is the use of strong drugs to treat cancer. You will often hear chemotherapy called "chemo," (key-mo) but it's the same treatment.*
Chemo was first used to treat cancer in the 1950s. It has helped many people live full lives. Research shows they work to help kill cancer cells (3)."

Here is what chemotherapy works, *"There are more than 100 chemo drugs used today. Doctors choose certain drugs based on the kind of cancer you have and its stage (how much cancer is in your body). Chemo can be used for different reasons. Your doctor will discuss these with you before you start treatment. Chemo may be used to keep the cancer from spreading; slow the cancer's growth; kill cancer cells that may have spread to other parts of the body; relieve symptoms such as pain or blockages caused by cancer; and cure cancer (3)."*

Now let's look at radiation and how it works, *"Radiation therapy uses special equipment to send high doses of radiation to the cancer cells. Most cells in the body grow and divide to form new cells. But cancer cells grow and divide faster than many of the normal cells around them. Radiation works by making small breaks in the DNA inside cells. These breaks keep cancer cells from growing and dividing, and often cause them to die. Nearby normal cells can also be affected by radiation, but most recover and go back to working the way they should.*

Unlike chemotherapy, which exposes the whole body to cancer-fighting drugs, radiation therapy is usually a local treatment. It's aimed at and affects only the part of the body being treated. The goal of radiation treatment is to damage cancer cells, with as little harm as possible to nearby healthy tissue.

Some treatments use radioactive substances that are given in a vein or by mouth. In this case, the radiation does travel throughout the body. But for the most part, the radioactive substance collects in the area of the tumor, so there's little effect on the rest of the body

(www.cancer.org/treatment/treatmentsandsideeffects/treatmenttypes/radiation/ understandingradiationtherapyaguideforpatientsandfamilies/understanding- radiation-therapy-how-does-radiation-therapy-work)." All of these treatments are "cures" but that does not mean that once the cancer is gone that it will not ever come back.

There is one last treatment I would like to take a look at. This treatment is not like the traditional treatments that I have already talked about. This treatment is from the holistic branch of medicine. The treatment I am referring to is marijuana. I did a search on the internet and came across this website: www.naturalnews.com/0460046_medical_marijuana_cancer_treatment.ht ml#. On this website there is an article called ***Marijuana-A cure for cancer? Written by Chris Sumbs.*** This what Chris writes about the evidence of marijuana being use as a treatment for cancer, *"Studies were recently completed by the California Pacific Medical Center in the San Francisco Bay area. The compound CBD was tested on animals with cancer as an alternative treatment. They found there was a disruption in the growth of tumors cells. CBD is a natural defense mechanism in the cannabis plant. In fact, CBD makes up about 40 percent of the cannabis plant matter. CBD is considered non-psychoactive, whereas THC is psychoactive. Basically, CBD doesn't give you the "high feelings" associated with THC, but it is showing promise in stopping or even reversing the effects of cancer on the body.*

By manipulating the breeding of the plants to achieve high contents of CBD and low content of THC, this could give a very low psychoactive response yet provide all the cancer fighting benefits of the CBD.

This breakthrough discovery is on the verge of being tested on humans with both brain cancer and breast cancer. If this works, marijuana could be the single biggest breakthrough treatment we've seen for cancer; perhaps ever!"

Chapter Three

I am sure that there a few a few people out there that believe that the poor are the only ones that are taken by the nasty disease called cancer. Cancer DOES NOT CARE whether you are rich or poor it will take your life just the same. There have been a ton of celebrities and famous people that cancer has taken as its own.

Let's take a look at some of the celebrities and famous people who have died from some form of cancer. The list is every long so I am going to shorten it a little. I will list the type of cancer they died from if I know it. So get comfortable because here it comes.

1. Nat "King" Cole (lung cancer)
2. Bette Grable (lung cancer)
3. Gary Cooper (lung cancer)
4. Walt Disney (lung cancer)
5. Yul Brenner (lung cancer)
6. Desi Araz (lung cancer)
7. John Wayne (lung cancer)
8. Jimmy Dorsey (lung cancer)
9. Donna Summer
10. Bea Arthur
11. Dom DeLuise
12. Dennis Hopper
13. Andy Kaufman
14. Peter Jennings (lung cancer)
15. Farrah Fewcett (anal cancer)
16. John Walker (liver cancer)
17. Patrick Swayze (pancreatic cancer)
18. Jack Benny (pancreatic cancer)
19. Donna Reed (pancreatic cancer)
20. Joan Crawford (pancreatic cancer)
21. Steve Jobs (pancreatic cancer)
22. Bill Hick (pancreatic cancer)
23. Gilda Radner
24. Bob Marley
25. Jacqueline Kennedy Onassis
26. Babe Ruth
27. Dizzy Gillespie (pancreatic cancer)
28. Morton Feldman (pancreatic cancer)

29. Fernando Lamas (pancreatic cancer)
30. Rex Harrison (pancreatic cancer)

The list goes on and on. I think I have made my point that cancer will claim whoever it wants to, be them rich; be them poor; be them celebrities or be them famous. It does not matter to cancer who you are if it wants you it WILL take you.

Cancer as even raised its ugly head in love ones close to me. When I say close I mean in my immediate family. Cancer decided to take one and spare the other. In the next two chapters I am going to tell you their stories.

Chapter Four

In this chapter I am going to tell you the story of Dad and his battle with cancer. I am going to start with his life. That is the parts of it that I know of. I write this in loving memory of my dad.

My dad was born on March 2, 1926. His parents gave him the Ewald James Rausch. He fought in World War II. He married my mom on November 4, 1946. They had nine children of which one died when she was two years old. This the back down of the ones of us that are still alive which is the remaining eight children. They had five girls and three boys.

What my dad lacked in money he made up in love and kindness. Growing up we were poor. My dad worked at the local pawn shop. I didn't see much of my dad growing up he work 12 hour shifts. He would get home after us kids went to bed and would still be a sleep when we got up to go to school. He worked seven days a week.

Even during summer vacation my dad had to work. We would go camping at the local lake every year. We would camp for two weeks during the summer. The whole time we were camping my dad had to work. He would have to drive into town to work and then he would return after work. I seem to remember seeing him more during summer vacation than any other time during the year.

I don't know if he made some kind of arrangement with his boss to be able to spend time with his family during our summer vacation. While we were camp we would play softball a lot. I can remember having so much fun during these camping trips. The whole family seemed to be having as much fun as I was. I know my dad really seemed to enjoy his time with his children.

Like I said earlier my dad worker at the local pawn shop. It was well he was working that he would show his kindness to strangers. When someone would bring in whatever they wanted to pawn my dad would check it out very carefully. Sometimes he would find in a pocket of a bag or suitcase. He wouldn't remove it he would simple ask the person if they are sure they want to pawn it and if they would say yes he would tell them to check all the pockets to make they didn't leave anything in them. The money that he would find was usually more than they would get if they pawned it. The person would check the pockets and find the money that my dad had found. They would end up not pawning it. They could thank my dad enough for alert them to the money. If he didn't find money he would give them a little more than the boss told him to. Again the people would be very thankful.

During the holidays young soldiers would come in to pawn their stuff because they wanted to have a good meal for the holidays. My dad would tell them to keep their stuff and he would invited them to our house for Thanksgiving or Christmas dinner. I cannot remember a time when there wasn't some stranger at our house eating with us on the holidays. Even though we didn't have much money ourselves he still shared these meals with these people. I honestly don't know how he afforded to feed these people unless he used his holiday bonuses to buy extra food.

My dad would help anyone if he could. It didn't matter if it was family, friends or strangers. I admired my dad for doing this. My dad was also mean when he had to be. Especially, when it came to someone mistreating one of his kids. My dad was the gentles man I knew until you pissed him off. If you ever pissed him off you had better run.

My dad was always there for me, probably more than he should have been. I knew that I could always go to him if I had a problem or needed something or needed help or if I just needed someone to talk to.

My dad has as long as I can remember tried to instill in his children to help each other when and if they can. He didn't like to hear or see his children fighting with each other. My dad would always tell us, "When your mother and I are gone you will only have each other." He would really get upset when heard of one of his children not help another when he knew they could have.

Back in 2006 my future wife, kids and myself was living in Lakewood, Colorado. One day I was on the computer surfing the web when my sister Donna messengered me to tell me that our dad was diagnosed with pancreatic cancer and that he was in the hospital. His doctor planned to go in and cut out all the cancer.

Hours later my sister got back to me and told me that his doctor said the surgery was a success. His doctor told my dad that he was able to get all of the cancer. That was very good news for the whole family. My dad went on to live a good life.

In 2008 my family and I moved back to Kansas. We visited my parent as often as we could. My dad started to whittle down to nothing. I mean this poor man couldn't eat anything that didn't go straight through him. One day while we were visiting my dad got up out of his chair to walk over to the window to see the van that we had bought. The poor man only took a few steps before he became dizzy and I had to get up to help him back to his chair. He told me that it happen a lot. He told me that his doctor didn't know why.

My family and I went back to Topeka where we lived at the time. Topeka is about an hour or so from Junction City where my parents lived. On the way home my wife told me that she had a very strong feeling that my dad was going to last long. She didn't know how right she was. The next morning I got a call from my sister Sue. She called to let me know that our dad was in the hospital because his cancer had come back with a vengeance.

I remember becoming sick to my stomach thinking of my dad's cancer coming back as fast strong that it did. I got off the phone and had to fight back the tears as I told my wife what my sister said. We got the kids read and hit the highway to go and visit my dad in the hospital. He looked terrible. His cancer was spreading quickly.

It wasn't long before his doctor decided that it was time for him to be moved back home to live out his last days. We would come down to spend time with him while the whole family waited for dreaded day that cancer would claim our dad. I hated seeing him like that. He was there but yet he wasn't. As much as I hated to I sat with him a while holding his hand and telling him how much I loved him.

While my dad was dying he would carry on conversations with his father and brother. The thing is they were both dead. They say this was normal because dying people usually see family members that are dead and talk to them. They say the dead family members come to help the one dying to make the transition.

Unfortunately, there was no room for us to stay in Junction City. Plus we didn't have the money to stay in a hotel so we had to travel back to Topeka. Thinking back it was fucked up because my sister Pam offered my son to stay with her but not my wife, her kids or me. Any way we went back to Topeka. We got the kids ready for bed and then my wife and I went to bed. I woke up to the phone ringing. I answered it and it was my sister Sue on the other end. She told me that our dad was dead.

I got off the phone in tears. My wife asked what was wrong and I told her that dad was dead. She started crying too. We got the kids ready as quickly as we could and headed to Junction City. We got to my parent's place. My mom told us that my dad was at the local funeral home and told me that I need to go view him. So, my wife and I went to the funeral home. They really did a good job to make my dad look good.

I felt extremely bad because I didn't get a chance to say good-bye to him before he died. I didn't say good-bye the day before because I was under the false belief that I had more time with him. I think it was the fact that I didn't want to let go of him. I tried to say good-bye while he was laying there on display. Guilt flowed over me like a waterfall because I waited too long to say good-bye. It just wasn't the same to say good-bye while laid there at least to me.

A few months after my dad's funeral I was in Junction City to visit my mom and she asked me to go visit my dad's grave. I told her I would so my wife, kids and I went to the cemetery. While I was there standing in front of his grave I tried once again to say good-bye to him. After saying my good-byes to my dad I started to feel better about it. I don't what was different about saying good-bye in the cemetery than when I said good-bye in the funeral home but whatever the reason it helped me to gain peace.

I bet you any amount of money that my dad is sitting up in heaven looking down on his children and crying, because we are farther apart now then we have been in forever. Some of us still talk to each other but others don't. To make things worse my mom isn't doing well at all. When she dies I believe that things between my siblings and I will only get worse.

Chapter Five

This chapter is going to be about my other love one that was diagnosed with cancer. That love one is my son. It really hard when you find out your dad has cancer but it is extremely harder when you are told your young son has cancer.

Back in 1992 I had a lot of stuff going on in my life. I was getting out of the Air Force. I was waiting for my divorce from my first wife. I was involved with my future second wife her name was Melody. I was traveling from North Dakota where I was stationed at the time to New Jersey where Melody's family lived. From New Jersey to Kansas for a family reunion. From Kansas back to New Jersey to visit some more. From New Jersey to Arizona where we were going to settle down.

While I was in New Jersey spending time with my new girl's family I got my final divorce papers in the mail. When I received the papers we had a celebration to say good-bye to the old and hello to the new.

I enjoyed my time with her family but it was time to get on the road to Arizona. The trip was long and interesting. We basically went from one coast to the other. Before heading to Arizona I sent my parents some money to get us a place. The plan was for my parents and us to share a place to live.

By the time we got to Arizona my parents had a place and everything hooked up. After getting to Arizona I had to make a trip to California to get my household goods out of storage. That is where I had the military ship my stuff because that is where I joined the military at. If I hadn't done it that way I was told they wouldn't pay for the move. I got my stuff with the help of my brother-in-law at the time to get my stuff moved to Arizona.

It took me a few months to find a job. I finally went to work across the river at a casino in Laughlin, Nevada. My job was to provide security for the casino. Melody eventually found a job in Laughlin too. She found a job at the same casino I was working at. She started out in a little jewelry booth and then she got a job at the ice cream shop that was in the casino.

At my three month mark at work I decided to marry Melody so she could be put on my insurance. We decided to make a trip to Las Vegas and went to one of those small wedding chapels on the side of the road. The place we went to was the same place that a lot of celebrities went to when they got married. Celebrities like Michael Jordan and Liz Taylor.

We were in Arizona for about one year before things started to change. Melody started to feel as though she couldn't do anything around the house. She said she would like to make dinner sometimes but she felt she couldn't. I asked her if she talked to my mom about it and she said no. I asked her how she knows she can't if she doesn't. Well she never did. Instead she wanted to move.

So, in early 1993 we made that move to North Carolina. We found a place to live and I found a job. I went to work for a warehouse. Melody got a job at the trailer park where we lived. My parents even decided to move into the trailer park too. When we decided to move left them without a place because they couldn't afford the place once we left. So, they packed up and we all went on the road and ended up in Charlotte, North Carolina.

My oldest brother Tim and his family lived in Charlotte as well. We visited with him for a little while before we decided to live there. In the middle of 1993 we decided to try to get pregnant which she did. On March 25, 1994 our son was born. We named him Jordan. He was the light of our lives.

I continued to work for the warehouse until Melody talked to a friend of ours that was working for a fire control company. He went around cleaning cooking hoods in delis and restaurants. He told her how much money he was making which was a whole lot more than I was at the warehouse. He told her he could get me a job. So she talked to me about and I agreed to change jobs.

Well it turned out badly because it turned out that I was making less than I was at the warehouse plus I was out of town more than I was in town. Our marriage started to suffer. We started growing apart. When I was in town we would go and do our own thing. We didn't do things together any more. So I went back to work at the warehouse. They were so glad to get me back. Thing took a turn for the worse, for reasons I am not going to state here she lost her job.

While all this was going on her father had died. So when she lost her job we decided to move to New Jersey to be closer to her mom. We lived with her mom for a while. Things continued to get bad in our marriage. It got to the point where we would hardly talk to each other. In fact when we decided to go our own ways we were sitting at the VFW bar. She was working there and I was sitting at the bar keeping her company.

Her mother was watching Jordan for us while we were at the VFW. At the time there wasn't anyone at the bar so we could have talked but instead we wrote notes back and forth. We couldn't even use our words to talk about this very important thing instead we decided to write it down. While we both agreed that our marriage wasn't working any more. In the letter we decided to separate. We also decided that it would be best for me to take Jordan because she said she had some things she needed to work out and she wanted to do it without worrying about taking care of a child.

I took Jordan and moved back to Junction City, Kansas. We moved in with my parents and my oldest sister Della. Thank goodness the house was a big one. I went to work at the footlocker distribution center. My divorce from Melody was final in 1997. I now moved into the world of being a single father. In the divorce I got residential custody of Jordan.

I worked for footlocker for a while before getting a job doing security on the Army Base just outside of town in 2003. I worked there for about a year when I met a girl her name was Deb. She worked at one of the strip clubs in town. It wasn't long before I decided to move in with her. The strange things was that she lived in Missouri. I don't know why she was working so far from home and I never asked.

While I was living with her Jordan developed a high fever one night. We took him to the emergency room to see why. It turned out that he had mono. They gave him some medication for it and he got over it. Things went well for a while between Deb and me but soon that all changed. It was like she had two different personalities. I never knew which personality I was going to get. Needless to say things didn't work out between the two of us and I ended up moving back to Kansas.

In 2005 I met my soul-mate. Her name is Astric. Like Forest Gump said, "We were like peas and carrots." We were a match made in heaven. I had seen her in 2004 and when I first laid eyes on her I said to myself that I was going to marry her someday. I didn't actually met her until 2005. It was love at first sight. The more I got to know her the more I knew we were meant to be together. She felt the same way.

In 2006 when we were living in Colorado and my dad was going through his battle with cancer Jordan came to Astric and me and said that he had a pea size bump in his neck. We told him we would keep an eye on it. Well it went away and he never said anything about it until 2007.

In 2007 during one weekend Jordan came to us again and said something about the pea size bump was back. We checked it out and told him once again that we would keep an eye on it. I had to go to work the next night. While I was at work the pea size bump in his neck grew to the size of a softball. Jordan was in terrific pain and he was in tears.

Astric called me at work and told me I needed to come home and take Jordan to the emergency room. She explained to me what was going on. I got off the phone with her and called my supervisor. I told him what was going on and that I needed to be relieved so I could take Jordan to the hospital. At first he wanted to argue with me about getting relieved. But about a half hour later someone was at my site relieving me.

I rushed home to get Jordan. While we were driving to the hospital I was trying to lighten the mood by joking around. So in my best Arnold Schwarenegger voice I used the line from his Terminator movie where he says, "I'll be back." I changed the words and said, "It's not a tumor." We both laughed a little. But later at the hospital I felt like an ass because it turned out to be a tumor.

We were at the emergency room for a few hours as they checked the lump out. Than they came in and told us that they were going to transfer him to another hospital that was better equipped to handle what he had going on. They put Jordan in an ambulance and I followed the ambulance to the new hospital. They got him all checked in and a doctor came in and told me that they were planning to operate and test the lump in his neck.

I got Jordan all settled in and then headed home to let Astric know what I found out. I told that the plan to test the lump to find out what it is. We all went to the hospital to spend time with Jordan before his surgery. After they wheeled him to the operating room we went and sat in the waiting area until his surgery was over. Once it was over one of the doctors came out and talked to us.

She told the operation went well and that they couldn't remove the tumor because it was too close to his carotid artery. Instead they took a piece of it and test it to find out that he had cancer. The type of cancer he was diagnosed with was Hodgkin Lymphoma. When the doctor told us that it felt like a sharp stick was shoved into our hearts. The last thing on earth that any parents wants to hear is that their thirteen year old child has cancer.

Once that doctor got done talking to us she told us that another doctor would be coming to talk to us more about it and the treatment plan. Astric and I both cried when we heard the news. The other doctor came out and told us more about it and that the plan was for him to go through chemotherapy. She told us that sometimes the mono virus can turn into cancer especially in boys.

Astric went back to the recovery room to see Jordan first. Jordan told her that it hurt mom. She visited with him for a little while then she came out and I went back to see him. When she came out she told me that she couldn't tell him that he had cancer. So when I went back to see him I couldn't bring myself to say the words, "You have cancer." All I could do is tell him that it is the worst case scenario. He said, "I have cancer" and tearfully I said yes.

He got to come home and it wasn't long before it was time to start his chemotherapy treatments. He had to go to the clinic get hooked up to IVs filled with the chemo. The treatments took about eight hours. He had to go through these treatments every two weeks. When he wasn't doing the liquid chemo he had to take thirteen pills every day. This went on for six months.

After each chemo treatment poor Jordan looked like death warmed over. The chemo also caused his hair to fall out. His immune system was shot after each chemo treatment. That mean he was pretty much left to being in the house all the time. He couldn't go to school because if he caught anything from another kid it could be deadly to him.

This meant he had to be home schooled. They school system would send a teacher to our house every day to teach Jordan. Some times after a treatment he would develop an infection which would develop into a high fever so he would have to go to the hospital so they could get his fever down.

The poor child had to have four blood transfusions. After his transfusion we all had to wear surgical marks so that he didn't caught anything from us. During these times he would stay in his room away from everyone.

It wasn't until he was almost down with his treatments that they finally figured out what was causing the fevers. They had put what they called a drug port in his chest and that how they administered the chemo. That is what was causing the fevers because his body was rejecting it.

After six months of chemotherapy and other cancer drugs his cancer went into remission. Thankfully it has stayed in remission to this day. Jordan will turn 21 this year (2015). Jordan is no longer living with Astric and me his now living with his mother and stepfather.

In 2007 not to long after Jordan was diagnosed with cancer Astric and I decided to get married. I am not completely sure why we waited until Jordan was diagnosed with cancer to finally take the next step and get married. I think she did it to let me know she wasn't going anywhere and to let me know she was in it for the long haul. Astric and I are still together to this day.

Chapter Six

Like I mentioned in chapter one there are a lot of organizations out there that collect money to help patients, their families and to fund research to find a cure. I would hope that you would think very carefully about reaching deep down into you pockets or purses and give to at least one of these organizations. If not to the ones I mentioned then please find one on your own and donate to it.

If it wasn't for these wonderful organizations that help a lot of cancer patients and their families would be left with nowhere to turn. I know if it wasn't for some of these organizations my family and I wouldn't have known what to do about how to get help paying our rent because my wife and I were both let go from our jobs. They just didn't understand why we had to miss a couple of days every two weeks.

If it wasn't for some of these organizations and others our children wouldn't have had a Christmas that year. But because of them our children had one of the best Christmas ever. They had so many presents to open that it took almost all Christmas day for them to open them all.

I want to take this time to thank some organizations again that helped us through this tough time. First and foremost I want to thank God for watching over Jordan and allowing him to survive cancer. I want to thank Cops Fighting Cancer. I want to thank There with Care. I want to thank the make a wish foundation of Colorado and Ozzy Osbourne who granted Jordan's wish. He got to go to Ozzy's concert in Denver and to meet him before the show. I want to thank the nurses at the clinic he did his chemo at for the stuff they did for us. I want to thank all the people that donated stuff to us when we did yard sales to raise money to help pay our bills.

Thank You for buying my book!!!!!!

Please don't forget to find a cancer organization to donate to!

Notes

1 google search, Mar. 7, 2014

2 google search, Feb. 4, 2013

3
www.cancer.org/treatment/treatmentsandsideeffects/treatmenttypes/chemo
theraphy/whatishowithelps/chemo-what-it-is-question-about-chemo.

4 google search, Feb.27, 2015

5
www.cancer.org/treatment/treatmentsandsideeffects/treatmenttypes/radiati
on/understandingradiationtherapyaguideforpatientsandfamilies/understand
ing-radiation-therapy-how-does-radiation-therapy-work.

6
www.naturalnews.com/040046_medical_marijuana_cancer_threatment.ht
ml#, Marijuana-A Cure for Cancer, April 24, 2013, Chris Sumbs.

www.ingramcontent.com/pod-product-compliance
Lightning Source LLC
Chambersburg PA
CBHW071347310526
45790CB00018B/1384